"The book is a prayerful experience. Each chapter begins with a quotation, cites a daily encounter, and ends with a prayer with the Lord as companion. It is a book that flows with the daily currents of life and sweeps one along. After reading it one has a tendency to bow one's head and say amen."

Anita Marie Howe, Ed.D.
Sisters of Charity of Cincinnati

"Margot writes with genuineness about the experience of being a pastor/chaplain. Her choice of materials is broad enough to interest any pastor. The commentary on her experiences visiting with the sick is refreshing and running over with valuable insight and inspiration. This is the kind of inspirational book any chaplain would do well to keep close at hand when the 'business' of ministry causes them to lose touch with the reason for answering their 'call.'"

Chaplain Donald F. Gum, FCOC
President, College of Chaplains

"*Caring for Yourself When Caring for Others* will be an important resource for persons engaged in caring for other people. Unless one attends to the needs of the self in proper ways, care for others will suffer. Care for the self involves spiritual, psychological, and physical discipline and requires understanding that it is not only all right, but mandatory if care for others is to be sustained.

"Margot Hover provides helpful, reflective chapters that can be used in a variety of ways. Together they make the case for disciplined self-care. They free the reader to think about the resentments and frustrations that are inevitable in caring for others. I hope that it will be read by parish clergy, seminarians, chaplains, nurses, and physicians. But the book will also be a real help to those involved in caring for others in a non-professional role: parents, spouses and children, especially when the need is acute. This volume deserves wide reading because it is theologically responsible, psychologically sophisticated, and spiritually appropriate."

Dennis M. Campbell
Dean of Divinity School and Professor of Theology
Duke University

"Hover's book provides a refreshing blend of scripture, life experience, and prayer from an experienced caregiver's perspective. This blend is essential if caregivers are to be effective in providing pastoral care for persons in crisis and if caregivers are to stay physically, emotionally, and spiritually alive in ministry.

"As I read the book, I felt like a peer walking with Margot. Her descriptions evoked both tears and laughter. This peer sharing is very important for pastoral caregivers who often walk alone. I would recommend the book for caregivers who want to share a journey with another caregiver."

Duane Parker, Ph.D.
Executive Director, Association for Clinical Pastoral Education

"The task of the care-giver is ever the quest for balance that is life-giving ...for the care-giver *and* the care-receiver. This is a balance between, on the one hand, not fostering dependency to the point of sacrificing the autonomy of the other person; and, on the other hand, not being so self-focused that one moves into a state of unhealthy narcissism.

"This book reflects Margot's understanding of the importance of that balance. Knowing Margot personally, I was particularly struck by her personal and professional growth at the point of keeping that balance in her own mothering and ministry. I was further touched by her vulnerability about her own dependency in her recent illness. In this book, Margot models for us all what she seeks to teach."

Rev. Leslie Young-Ward
Director of Clinical Pastoral Education
Birmingham, Alabama

"'Take a good look!' This is the invitation offered in *Caring for Yourself When Caring for Others* by Margot Hover. This refreshing, insightful, and supportive volume looks at those in need of care, those who care for them (chaplains, pastoral caregivers, lay ministers, eucharistic ministers). It is a collection of reflections/essays that open with Scripture and close with a brief prayer. Yet you never feel that religion is being forced on your attention. I felt that I was seeing myself, my feelings, my pain, my experiences, my questions, my longings. The book is a mirror to help me touch the things I must continue to touch if I am to continue my ministry.

"Hover is a great teacher for ministers of care (especially the many who are 'drafted' by religious communities and sent out, often with little training and even less support), and a gift of faithful support that all of us need in pastoral work."

Rev. Richard B. Gilbert, FCOC
Director of Pastoral Services
Valparaiso, Indiana

"Margot Hover's book is a gem! The essays provide a special form of understanding and support for caregivers. Filled with warmth and colored by humor, her reflections are a source of renewed hope and strength for all of us."

Andre Auw, Ph.D.
Co-Founder, Center for Studies of the Person

"Required reading for Clinical Pastoral Education students, this is an excellent companion for anyone working in health care—physicians, nurses, housekeepers, social workers, volunteers—in addition to chaplains. The style is easy, realistic, and frames the job of care-giving in the larger perspective of scripture and prayer. Read one passage a day—over lunch, on a break, when you get home from work—to put your job, feelings, and life back in proper order. It is what we need for attitude adjustment."

Rev. Chuck Meyer
Author, *Surviving Death*

"When Margot Hover shared with me excerpts from her *Caring for Yourself When Caring for Others*, I recognized that doctors and other health professionals would profit from reflecting on her simple (not simplistic), moving tales. These are important meditations for everyone confronted with the demands and rewards of caring for others. And who isn't?

"I commend her book to readers in general. Hover has put into action the good intention that so many of us have, but just never quite get around to doing: examining life and demonstrating how we can make it worth living. We profit from what she has seen and heard and thought and, perhaps, we can learn from her the habit of prayerful reflection on the daily events of our lives. It is no mystery why Jesus talked in parables instead of philosophical discourse: because storytellers change lives, while philosophers only change opinions. My thanks to Margot Hover for capturing in words those fleeting stories that she has formed into her book. We are all the better for it."

Francis A. Neelon, M.D.
Associate Professor of Medicine
Editor, *North Carolina Medical Journal*

"Caring for others can be debilitating if the care-giver does not take time to listen to herself and reflect on how to manager her own needs. *Caring for Yourself When Caring for Others* provides simple ways of listening and reflecting on the interaction between the care giver, care receiver, and others. It gives insight into the daily occurrences of life and the many little things that can support the care giver. The author draws on her own experiences of being both a care giver and a care receiver, pointing out that by listening and reflecting a mutuality of shared humanity is achieved.

Caring

FOR YOURSELF
WHEN
CARING FOR OTHERS

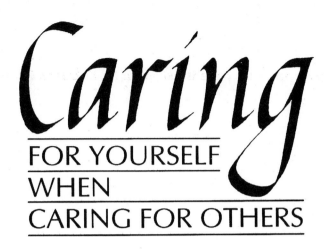

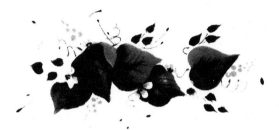

MARGOT HOVER

XXIII
TWENTY-THIRD PUBLICATIONS
Mystic, Connecticut 06355

Cover and title page illustration by Kathleen Lamb

Twenty-Third Publications
185 Willow Street
P.O. Box 180
Mystic CT 06355
(203) 536-2611
800-321-0411

ISBN 0-89622-533-X
Library of Congress Catalog Card Number 92-60890

Foreword

Caring for Yourself When Caring for Others is a spiritual journey of twenty-five steps through which every minister walks over a certain period of time, or perhaps even daily. It is a journey in which ministerial activities and other happenings in life confront us with our limitations and the need for a deeper meaning. This daily confrontation with our human self and our call to reach out to others bring home the necessity to find the underlying reasons for our own being and vocation.

Margot Hover guides us on this journey. She opens with a "wake-up call" that points out that our ministry is unsuccessful without God's continuous presence. Then she takes us through three stages:

1. Coming to grips with the awareness of the insufficiency of our "outward activity." This is highlighted in step four when she experiences that patients do not always follow the book and seem to upset our effectiveness as ministers.

2. Searching for an integration of spiritual values into everyday life and ministry. She shows it in step six when she discovers the importance of "small talk" with patients, and in step seven when she sees the need to understand *the cause* of the patients' fear or denial.

3. Actively integrating daily life with a meaning beyond its external appearance, as in step ten where she says (or prays), "I know that God is with me even in the frazzled times." But

this process has its ups and downs. Sometimes we need an external sign or symbol that God is really with us, as in step fourteen; other times we need to sit back and allow the meaning of certain events to roll over us and to penetrate the defenses of our activities and expectations.

Every step ends with a prayer that summarizes her search and efforts to integrate a spiritual presence in daily ministry. By this integration Margot makes us more deeply aware of the meaning and value of ministry. By accepting our "humanness," it becomes easier to live with it, to reach beyond it, and to minister with the wholeness of our being.

Cornelius J. van der Poel, C.S.Sp.
Director, Health Care Ministry Program
Barry University

Contents

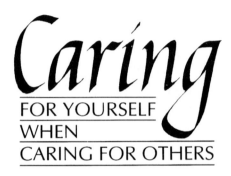

Caring

FOR YOURSELF
WHEN
CARING FOR OTHERS

Introduction

Sometimes caregiving "ain't all it's cracked up to be." Thomas Merton wrote, "Prayer and love are really learned in the hour when prayer becomes impossible and your heart turns to stone."

Caregivers know many of those moments. There comes a time when the old truism, "It's good to be needed," wears thin, and our world seems full of neediness that can't be fixed. Those times come to caregivers of all kinds: parents, health care workers, family members of the sick or disabled, parish ministers to the sick. The morning after a particularly trying evening, I ruefully told a sympathetic co-worker, "I knew rearing these kids might be the most important thing I might do with my life, but I didn't know it would be the *last* thing." A mother herself, she nodded with real empathy. On the bus ride home, an elderly neighbor who cares for her bedridden husband confessed, "I feel so bad when I get curt and impatient sometimes at the end of the day." My role as a parish Minister of the Eucharist is a very important part of my spirituality and vision of the church. Most of the time, I am energized by my visits to the sick...until that lovely Sunday afternoon when everyone else is at the beach and the tabernacle key isn't where it's supposed to be.

These chapters address those moments. I've come to think of this book as a look at the underside of the diamond of caregiving, an examination of the facets that usually don't show. The following chapters, borrowing Jesus' metaphor for ministry, are signposts for shepherds in the far pasture. May these reflections help to nurture and sustain you in your work of providing companionship, counsel, and consolation to those you care for.

Supporting His Hands

When your helping hand grows tired

> Moses' hands, however, grew tired; so they put a rock in place for him to sit on. Meanwhile, Aaron and Hur supported his hands, one on one side and one on the other, so that his hands remained steady till sunset.
>
> Exodus 17:8-13

Remember this story? One of the many adventures of the Jewish people in the desert was a battle with Amalek. Joshua did the fighting, but Moses evidently controlled the outcome by standing on a nearby hill with the staff of God upraised in his hand. When he lowered his arms, the battle turned against the Hebrews; they fared better when he raised his arms again.

What power! What responsibility! What a temptation for caregivers, to feel that the outcome for a sick child, spouse, or parent, or for a hospitalized parishioner is entirely in our hands. "If we had only noticed his symptoms earlier, perhaps we could have caught it sooner," we second guess ourselves. "If I hadn't left him alone...." "If I had given her the right vitamins...." "If we had only insisted that he quit that stressful job...." "If I had only brought Communion to him as soon as he called...."

How often second guessing ourselves is an attempt to regain a sense of control over events that are essentially out of our control. Somehow we think that accepting blame is less painful than admitting that some things simply just happen, without our help and despite our best efforts. Human bodies are both amazingly intricate and disconcertingly fragile. Mothers who watched every morsel they ate during pregnancy give birth to babies with birth defects. Adults who exercise and diet conscientiously have heart attacks and strokes. The difficult truth is that our battles are much less predictable than the one the Hebrews fought with Amalek. And that, in the final analysis, may be the most difficult reality to accept.

It's the other half of the story that gives us hope. When Moses grew tired, Aaron and Hur helped him by finding a rock for him to sit on and supporting his uplifted arms as they grew tired. Where are the Aarons and Hurs in your life?

A recent newspaper advice column included a reader's diatribe against what has become a standard greeting, "Have a nice day." The letter writer assumed that people uttered that blessing mindlessly, and so she took grave offense. I read the feature as I rode the bus to work; when I put the paper down, I became aware of the conversations around me. People who knew each other only because they usually met the bus at the same stop each day were comparing notes on what they did the preceding evening, what they anticipated during that day's work, and how they planned to spend their vacations. Hands were extended to assist a passenger who was loaded down with dishes for a noontime potluck. Attention and sympathy were showered on a woman wearing a new foot-brace after a fall the day before. "Have a good day," called the passengers as they disembarked, to which the driver responded, "You too." To be honest, I was a bit surprised at how much that warmth, shared among relative strangers, meant at the beginning of my day. I began paying attention to the smiles I received from strangers I passed in the hallways, and to the exchanges of recognition and warmth in routine telephone calls. Small symbols of support, admittedly. But then, so was supporting Moses' arms, on the surface of it.

What small gifts appear in the moments of your daily routine as a caregiver? The flicker of a smile on the face of someone who is usually critical or unresponsive? The greeting of the mailman? A moment's respite to muse at the kitchen window? Ten minutes to spend with a good book before drifting off to sleep at night?

I wonder if we don't sometimes let those small nurturing moments go by unnoticed and unappreciated in our dissatisfaction with the difficulty in finding large amounts of support—a neighbor's offering a whole Saturday's respite care, for instance. After all, what a "small" contribution Aaron and Hur made...to the winning of the war.

Dear Jesus, your life on earth was filled with "little things": seaside breakfasts of fresh fish, lilies of the field and birds of the air, dinner with friends like Mary, Martha, and Lazarus, soothing foot baths, sips of cold water from an unlikely new friend at the well. I know that those moments are present in my life, too, to nourish and sustain me. But when I'm tired or overworked, it is difficult to recognize and enjoy them. Today, I give you thanks for these special gifts, and I ask your help in remaining open to them. Amen.

2

Fell to the Ground

When you cry so hard you laugh

> Paul continued speaking until midnight....Eutychus, who
> was sitting in the window, began to sink off into a deep
> sleep while Paul talked still longer. Overcome by sleep,
> he fell to the ground three floors below and was picked
> up dead. Acts 20:7-12

It's crazy, the things people find funny. Certainly, our first response to this story is shock. After all, the young man was
killed in his fall from the synagogue window. Evidently the
congregation was shocked, too. We imagine that Paul's disciples interrupt their discussion to rush to the child, and we
can picture their horror when they discover that the boy is
dead. Paul, always practical and never one to waste words or
time, resuscitates the boy. Then he turns on his heels, heads
back upstairs for a quick supper, and continues his conversation until dawn.

Serious as that story is, it has precipitated grins and guffaws
for countless pastors in touch with their own tendency toward
verbosity. And among long-suffering parishioners, there are
certain to be those sleepy souls who are grateful that they may
slide down in the pew or onto a neighbor's shoulder rather
than out of a third-floor window.

Like the blend of tragedy and comedy in the story, humor in
the universe of the sickroom takes on a unique character.

Incongruity, surprise, and silliness are inextricable from daily life. And because daily life for a shut-in or hospital patient is different in some ways from the workaday world, humor in this arena looks different, too.

Children know this intuitively. I used to serve as chaplain to a children's cancer unit, where the pint-sized patients decorated their IV poles with streamers, then rode them down the halls like scooters. When the children lost their hair with their chemotherapy, they kept their heads warm with an amazing variety of bonnets, caps, and wigs. Each child eventually discovered the possibilities for self-expression and creativity. The older children used their caps as mobile billboards where they displayed comic buttons and stickers; the younger patients pinned polka dots and other trimmings to theirs. Visitors were sometimes aghast that badges of such a dread disease were treated with such ease and silliness. "Doesn't she know she has cancer?" one asked. Her temptation was to mistake the humor there with lack of awareness or denial. In actuality, the children's fun was an expression of their acceptance of their cancer, and their determination to experience all facets of the life available to them in the hospital. "All facets" included pain, isolation, lack of control...and humor.

Sometimes, in the midst of our cares and our caretaking, we feel guilty or frivolous when we joke or laugh heartily. Friends are eager to lend a shoulder if we are sad, and they frequently tout the benefits of "having a good cry." But it is certainly equally important to give ourselves permission to have a good laugh at a funny joke or an incongruous occurrence, even in the midst of very tense or sad situations. Buddha is often represented laughing heartily. This deity is reverenced for his calm openness to *all* facets of life, joy and seriousness included. Like him, we can let ourselves experience all the feelings of each moment beyond artificial limits around what is " fitting."

Dearest Companion, you laughed with children...rested with the apostles...partied with Zacchaeus...as well as mourned at Lazarus's tomb...shook with fear at the premonition of your own death. We thank you for the moments of laughter and flashes of humor that bring relief and lightness to us on days that are sometimes heavy and dark with tension. Amen.

3

Nothing New
Under the Sun

When you feel blindsided by your own emotions

What has been is what will be, and what has been done is
what will be done; there is nothing new under the sun.
Ecclesiastes 1:9

Nearly five years ago, a good friend of mine died very suddenly and unexpectedly. We lived in different cities, and I suppose
I had taken her so for granted that I was startled at the grief
that overwhelmed me when I received word of her death. I
talked to our mutual friends and contributed to the memorial
rituals, and gradually, the ache of her absence subsided. I grew
accustomed to not writing to her or visiting her as I once regularly did. Until the other day.

I thought of my friend and was once more filled with the
sad emptiness I experienced when she died. I thought I han-
dled all that *then*, five years ago, I told myself. Which of
Kübler-Ross' stages of grief did I omit or slide through that
they should reach out to grab me now, after all this time?

What I gradually realized was that grief—and other feelings

as well—aren't events to be experienced or tasks to be completed once and for all. Losses set off a sequence of experiences. As time passes, we move through our feelings about the initial moment many times, each time from a different perspective or place in life. "I felt some of the old sadness when I came here today," said the father of a little boy who had died of cancer a year earlier, on his return to the hospital for a support group meeting. "But today I realized that I didn't still automatically look in the direction of Bobby's old room expecting to see him there." The pain of having lost a son was still there, and always will be, to some degree. But it looked a bit different from the vantage point of a year later.

Sometimes that's a mixed comfort. We'd like to think that we can *do* something about painful feelings, or that we can do something about them so well that they will go away once and for all. Or we may be reluctant to give up our grief. "I'm afraid that if I don't mourn anymore, it will be as though he never existed," said one recent widow. Some sects believe that the souls of those who die linger near their earthly homes, tied there by the grief of those they left behind. In a sense, they are released as their loved ones move through some of their sadness. But that concept itself implies also that our grieving somehow keeps the dead person "alive." Giving up one's grief means losing our loved one a second time.

Whatever grief means to us, or however we understand the grief process, it may be reassuring to view it in terms of a spiral, where we encounter or view those feelings many times, each time from a different vantage point. That's different from the linear view, where one climbs out of one's feelings, and where their return is viewed as a kind of backsliding. Emotions don't get "finished"; they visit us many times, each time at a different level.

Dearest Friend, there are today for me a host of feelings that have caught me almost without warning. I'd prefer to shed my tears once and for all, and have them over and done with. I'd love to claim for myself all those "good" stages like "integration" and "acceptance," but there I am again, angry or despairing, discouraged or impatient. Please help me to remember that you are always with me, even when it seems to me that I am in the far pasture in the dark by myself. Amen.

4

The Better Part

When you can't—and shouldn't—heal others' pain

> But the Lord answered her, "Martha, Martha, you are worried and distracted by many things; there is need of only one thing. Mary has chosen the better part, which will not be taken from her."   Luke 10:41-2

"When mom was diagnosed, someone gave me Elisabeth Kübler-Ross' book *On Death and Dying* to read. Some of her points fit how Mom was behaving, but most of them didn't. I keep telling Mom she should be angry, but she says, "What's to be angry about?"

The past few years have seen a burgeoning of information on various human feelings and processes. Death, grief, family functioning, abuse, interpersonal communication models—all have become the focus of research, books, TV programs, support groups and movements. One benefit of the popularity and accessibility of these materials is that people no longer label themselves and others as crazy or bizarre quite so easily. For instance, we've come to expect toddlers and teens to rebel, retirees to be ambivalent about their new "freedom," and the terminally ill or newly disabled to be angry or depressed.

In knowing more about how people *may* feel and react, however, we have come dangerously close to assuming that they *should* respond in those ways. Like Martha, we are "busy about many things," including how others feel. The unfortunate result is that we as caretakers begin to see ourselves as orchestrating others' processes. We assume that we have failed if they don't move through Kübler-Ross' stages of grief, for example—and in proper sequence and on time. I've listened to the sadness and regret of nurses and physicians when they've been unable to lead terminally ill patients to become angry over their situation. I've heard their frustrations, when, despite their most direct and insistent confrontations, parents of critically ill children persistently talk in terms of "When she gets well..." and "When we take him home..." despite the odds against such a happy outcome. The same nurse who says, "Of course, I knew I couldn't keep him from dying," adds in the next breath, "but I wonder what I should have said to get him past his denial."

The most obvious difficulty with this stance is that it usurps people's right to their own feelings and their unique ways of expressing those feelings. One of my keenest recollections of grief came during one late night shift as I was pastoring the large family of an elderly and beloved matriarch who had just died. There were, of course, tears and embraces of support, those more easily recognized and socially acceptable expressions of sadness. In the midst of that, however, one son-in-law wailed, "There ain't never going to be any more Apple Brown Betty." His statement was a profound, unique, and intensely personal way of expressing his loss, although it hardly fit any clinical script.

The second problem in seeing ourselves as directing the grieving process of those we care for is that this stance cuts us off from sharing in and being instructed and enriched—like Mary—by the process through which they do move. I listened to the mourner that night and offered my acceptance and comfort. But I've listened to that memory countless times since; it has taught me how to grieve losses in my own life, and has enabled me to cry over things that "the books" might deem insignificant or inappropriate or irrelevant. Perhaps it has made me more sensitive to the importance of the "little things" that I might otherwise have passed over in my rush to honor the "big" or "right" events, realities, or feelings. Put another way, maintaining a certain attention to and reverence for those we minister to and care for will enrich our experience vocabulary for dealing with our own inevitable losses of independence, of belonging, of self-sufficiency, of relationships in their current form, and of earthly life itself. In that sense, if we are open to this, we are ministered to by those we serve.

Dear Lord, you teach hard lessons. Please be with me as I struggle to listen carefully and sensitively to your presence in those I serve and care for, and to your instructions for me as they emerge in their lives and struggles. Sometimes circumstances occupy me with Martha's role. After all, someone has to pay the bills, make out the schedule, arrange for transportation, coverage, trips to the drug store...and so on. As gently as you affirmed Mary's quiet listening, lead me to tolerate those times when I can listen to your voice in the words of those I serve, especially when I give up my control and expectations of what they should say. You know how difficult that sometimes is for me. Amen.

5

A New Song

When you don't know where to turn

I waited and waited for you, Yahweh! Now at last you
have turned to me and heard my cry for help. You have
lifted me out of the horrible pit, out of the slough of the
marsh; you set my feet on a rock and steadied my steps.
Yahweh, you have put a new song in my mouth—a song
of praise. Many will look on in awe and will put their
trust in you.   Psalm 40*

In the area of psychology and the development of helping
skills, it was certainly people like Carl Rogers and Elisabeth
Kübler-Ross who taught us about the richness of trusting people "where they're at," as the saying goes. Rogers proved with
his clients the efficacy of reflective listening, focusing on what
his patients were telling him instead of concentrating on hidden meanings and patterns he found in their words. Kübler-
Ross often trusted her patients to know more about what was
happening within them than the doctors who based their pre-
dictions on such concrete and seemingly indisputable evidence
as lab results. So there is a good deal of evidence supporting
the stance that the best approach to those we would like to
help is to listen to them.

---

*Nancy Schreck, OSF and Maureen Leach, OSF, *Psalms Anew* (Winona, Minn.: St.
Mary's Press, 1986).

I've reflected on the possibility that a similar stance might be helpful in our relationship with God. Intense as I tend to be, I've spent a good portion of my spiritual life digging away to see who God is for me, and what God is working on in particular situations. I was relating my dedicated plugging away on this theme with a spiritual director one day, when she interrupted me with, "Why not let God do some of the work?" She stopped me in my tracks. What an incredibly novel idea, I thought. But what if...my mind raced ahead to alternative plans, in case God were silent beyond my tolerance for that? It required no small measure of self-control to stop my frantic activity, to "rest in the Lord."

I remember years ago hearing about an Eskimo sculptor who always began his work on a fresh chunk of soapstone by pausing and asking, "I wonder what shape is hiding here in this stone." He saw his art as a process of listening to the whispered message of the figure that already rested in the raw material, and which would emerge only to the extent that he was able to gently and patiently wait for its instructions about how it might be liberated. Preconceived ideas about what *he* wanted to create merely got in the way of the stone spirit's work to reveal and unveil itself.

Thus, his artistry resided not in his skill with hammer and chisel, but in his finely honed ability to wait and to listen, probably even occasionally to tolerate the silence.

Of course, that suggests other problems. What if the message that I hear is not what I wanted? As long as I am working at top intensity to find God's word to me, I have a good deal of control over what I hear—whether it is God's word or the echo of my own. Listening quietly for the spirit within the stone or the word of God within daily events is not easy. It is an art.

Assuming this stance in my role as helper means that I become a recipient as well as a provider of care. My life is enriched by the insights others share, and my vision is challenged by the perspective from which they speak. Today, I visited two head and neck cancer patients, who, knowing that the usual treatments for their disease had failed, were now volunteering for an experimental chemotherapy. I expected them to talk about their fears or their anger or a number of other feelings associated with this kind of illness and death. Instead, as we prayed together, both shared tears of joy over their deep sense of God's abiding love and care for them. They were sensitive to the small evidences—a relative's phone call, a dietician's smile, warm blankets, or a favorite dish on the supper tray—things I regularly overlook when I'm busy searching for God in my life.

I thought of those visits when I picked up my nine-year-old son from his after-school program several days later. "I've been thinking," he began as soon as I shut the car door. "Why is it that God isn't talking to us these days? I haven't heard from him in a long time." Today, God spoke to me in words I could not miss, spoken most clearly by those I serve.

Dearest God, you spoke to the prophets and kings and to ordinary folks like us in ordinary ways so much of the time...even your Son looked like us. Remind us to listen without panic for your voice to sound loud enough for us to hear, and give us the confidence that you will speak, that the frightening, lonely silences that sometimes surround us are only the prelude to your more easily discerned voice of comfort and support. Amen.

6

Like Trees Walking

When you wonder what is really important

...When he had put saliva on his eyes and laid his hands on him, he asked him, "Can you see anything?" And the man looked up and said, "I can see people, but they look like trees, walking."   Mark 8:23,24

In our work of giving care, we generally focus on the feelings and needs of the recipient. As a parent, I ask about my son's day (and conduct) when I pick him up each evening. I open each pastoral visit by asking how the patient is doing. When I call my elderly mother, I expect that she will share with me the details of her week's activities and the outcomes of her doctors' visits. This, I've generally assumed, is the way caregiving goes.

Until the other day, when the tables tilted, if not turned, on me. My doctor found a "shadow" lurking in a routine x-ray, taken prior to very minor surgery. That set off three days of exhaustive and exhausting tests. Radiologists looked worried, and technicians patted my shoulder as they spoke of "masses" and colostomies.

Ultimately, the "shadow" disappeared, at least temporarily; my wry explanation was that it wore out. In the whole process, however, my universe warped and twisted like a fun-house mirror. I had already wearied of my self-absorption prior to the planned minor surgery, with half of my energy seeping away in anxiety and the other half going toward arranging for my household to function smoothly with a minimum of my involvement. Suddenly, it looked as though I might not be involved at all, at least for a while. My self-absorption intensified.

My memory of those days of tests is that, while my body took deep breaths and held them when it was told to by technicians, my mind frantically created its own world where my despair and my anger at God—what God!—wove through contingency plans for my family. The intensity of my dwelling in that world was so great that, when I returned to home and work, I was completely disoriented, like the blind man of the Gospel. I felt alien, and was almost surprised to notice that my co-workers were speaking the same language as I. I was slow in returning to the "normal" world once more.

Now, as I bring that experience into who I am as a pastoral caregiver, I remember that isolation and alienation. Like the man born blind, I re-entered the world of the well with confusion. I remember wishing for a good chaplain who could listen patiently and sensitively, of course. But my new realization was that I wanted someone who would connect me with the world outside myself and outside the Radiology Department, rather than focusing solely on me and my feelings.

Make no mistake about it. I know the difference between reassuring conversation that re-connected me with the world of friends and colleagues, and the babbling of those who "didn't know what to say." In fact, I struggled with that myself, as I tried to help those who looked as though they wanted to reach out to me. Some—those who were afraid of me—babbled nervously, in a frightening parody of my own fear. The others sat with me, held my hand, asked how I was, then told me how my students were doing in my absence, how my hospital unit was progressing, and how the office had received messages of concern. That the weather had turned cold reminded me that there was a world outside my own internal world of anxiety. Staff meeting gossip evoked images of reassuring patterns. There was no such thing as "small talk," only conversation that pushed me away or drew me back into comforting routine.

That experience has made me look differently at my own pastoral conversations with those I serve. I used to be very cautious about small talk, generally assuming that there were more important things to share in those situations. Not so, I now know.

My Comforter, you who have chosen me to minister to others both in my professional work and in my personal life, help me not to be afraid. Sometimes my anxiety about appearing awkward or insensitive or my fear of the lessons I might hear from those I serve stands like a barricade between us. Help me to honor the value of those pleasantries that bring us together in the fabric of the life we share as your people. Amen.

7

A Building from God

When you explore your own belief system

For we know that if the earthly tent we live in is destroyed, we have a building from God, a house not made with hands, eternal in the heavens.   2 Corinthians 5:1

Perhaps it's just me. I may be simply morbid. Or perhaps working with dying folk for so many years has helped me to follow along, if not head into, pastoral conversations about death. When recently faced with the possibility that my own life might be foreshortened, I quickly moved to plan for the details of that eventuality in a way that felt realistic to me rather than avoidant. After all, as a single parent of a young son, I knew what I had to do; as chaplain to many patients who shared my suspected diagnosis, I had a fairly clear picture of how long I had to do it in.

I wasn't so comfortable with the "after that." For years, I had spoken of hospital ministry as a matter of accepting the invitation to be instructed by those dealing with various aspects of the fragility of life. I realized that I had listened better to their fear, anger, denial, and acceptance than to their insights about *what* they were accepting. I also became acutely aware that I had generally avoided that topic in my own praying and reflecting. Death had become nearly an end in itself rather than the means to an end.

Now that the crisis of the moment has passed for me, I find myself relieved that I do not have to answer that question, "Where is life ultimately headed?" right now. Still, it seems like an important question, so I reluctantly hold myself to looking at it in somewhat the same way I address the task of the week's ironing. If I don't do it now, I'll need the answer unexpectedly one day, and it won't be ready.

A second event that precipitated my relative urgency to figure out what I believe about an afterlife was a pastoral visit to an end stage melanoma patient and his wife. She, Catholic, said wryly but emphatically, "I certainly don't believe in little heads with wings flying around heaven. But I told our daughter, 'God is taking Daddy because he ran out of angels and needed some new ones.'" Her formerly Anglican husband said quietly and reflectively that his belief in God and an afterlife diminished as he reflected on world tragedies and injustices, as well as on what seemed like the injustice of his own death.

Together, we forged a vocabulary that enabled each to feel the other's support amid their struggle to understand what was happening. Meanwhile, I went back to my old standby, Chardin's vision of the Omega point, where the Christification of the universe will ultimately occur. Chardin's framework has long provided me with a helpful image of the continuity of life. Still, I listen intently as dying patients tell me about their sense of going to rest or reward or reunions. I listen...and wonder.

So, God, who are you really, in the end? How do I hold onto the tangible images of my future for comfort and reassurance, amid my awareness that words and images cannot capture this unknown at all? Amen.

8

Went Away Grieving

When your care has been rejected

Jesus said to him, "If you wish to be perfect, go, sell your possessions, and give the money to the poor, and you will have treasure in heaven; then come, follow me." When the young man heard this word, he went away grieving, for he had many possessions.

Matthew 19:21,22

It was one those moments that for a long time afterward I could remember only with chagrin. Each Thursday, staff and students would visit a patient together. In rotation, one would select the patient and another would interview, with the rest joining in at the end of the visit and again as the group processed the experience later. It was my turn to conduct the pastoral visit, and the profile the presenter provided was so heartbreaking that I swept into the hospital room with the others in tow prepared to offer compassion and empathy pressed down and running over. Despite the patient's earlier enthusiastic consent to the visit, he took one look at me and pulled the sheets up tightly over his head. After I issued several gentle, albeit embarrassed, invitations to the unyielding form on the bed, we had no choice but to retreat.

As my embarrassment before my peers and students subsided, I began to reflect on the positive value of rejection in the context of pastoral relationships. When I thought about it, I realized that the chaplain is almost certainly the only person a hospital patient can safely refuse. While the Patient Self-determination Act has made us all aware that we should not approach end-of-life decisions passively, most other decisions for patients in hospitals and other care facilities either have painful implications or are made by others. If a patient consistently refuses to eat, he may be placed on IVs or tube feedings. "Routine" tests and treatments don't come buffet style; doctors select and order them and patients generally comply. Choices like whether to submit to chemotherapy or not come with such huge consequences that they almost don't seem like choices. So in retrospect, I saluted this patient's ability to seize the opportunity to make a clear and unequivocal statement about what he didn't want.

Much later on, when I myself was needy, I saw the risk he took in refusing our care. Independence comes with some costs and fears. For instance, if I refuse this offer now, will it come again when I feel differently about it? And can folks be connected without being needy? Parishioners may willingly go to the grocery for a homebound elder; would they as willingly stop by just for a cup of coffee and a chat? Or would I have visited this patient if his story had been less dramatic?

Dear Lord, being a pastor—opening doors and taking the first step toward others—is hard, as when my hand is pushed aside or I have to bear the burden of a pastoral conversation without much response. Give me the courage to continue, and the wisdom to be faithful to those I serve amid their own valuable freedom to respond. Amen.

9

All the Work by Myself

When your "virtue" becomes a vice

But Martha was distracted by her many tasks; so she came to him and asked, "Lord, do you not care that my sister has left me to do all the work by myself? Tell her then to help me."   Luke 10:40

It's strange and a bit alarming how seductive self-sacrifice can become. Especially to parents and professional caregivers. I noticed, for example, that I take a perverse kind of pride in how little time I may set aside for myself during a busy weekend of my son's basketball games, housecleaning, errands, and church work. Even when I began feeling better during a recent six-week convalescence, it felt risky to say aloud, "Great Scott! I'm loving every minute of this leisure. It's truly heavenly!" Eric Berne would label this playing the "Harried" game, and it comes all too naturally to those of us who operate under the illusion that we daily earn our salvation.

To be honest, opportunities for huge helpings of leisure or luxury, self-indulged or bestowed by others, may not often appear on our plates. After all, reality does reign, duty does call, and baby needs shoes. Nevertheless, I have begun wondering if "virtue" isn't sometimes its own punishment. That line of reflection led me one recent Lent to repent—re-think—my habits of self-sacrifice. I resolved to identify and zestfully claim some of the moments that I enjoy, that renew my spirit and make me easier to live with, as well. I share here a selection from my current list of re-creative moments and activities in the hope that it may spark your own re-thinking.

First, in a hospital environment that requires frequent energetic handwashing, I began using hand lotion. It feels and smells good, and the application process affords me a few moments to think about one visit before I begin another. Sometimes I pray, as I massage healing lotion into my fingers. Sometimes I look around me with renewed keenness. Sometimes I let my mind and feelings rest. Mostly I enjoy.

At our hospital, one can shortcut from one building to the other through a parking garage which is dark, full of fumes and squealing cars. Or one can take a path between the garage and a large rock garden terrace, landscaped with trees and flowers that provide color in all seasons. I suspect the two paths are the same length; perhaps one seems more earnest than the other. I take the garden path.

Can we really talk! I usually buy my lipsticks from the display at the grocery checkout lane. This year, I got one from a department store cosmetic counter.

This year, I did *not* have a garden. I think my previous custom dated to the 1960s when I collected seed catalogues each spring, and canned anything that sat still long enough. My yearly idealism got me through tilling and planting, but not through weeding. Truthfully, I like sitting in the sun with a glass of iced tea much more.

While I love watching my son play basketball and baseball, I'm not much of a sports fan. I do enjoy needlework and writing in my journal. Now I take them with me to games, and we both have a good time.

I take my lunch time seriously. Most days, I look at the stack of projects on my desk and think it would be better to tackle them while I eat my sandwich in my office. But emergencies aside, I generally either go for a walk outside or meet friends. On Fridays, I join an interdisciplinary group that discusses poetry and short stories dealing with medical themes. That I return energized to my work is the "icing on the cake." Now, you're on your own to build your list. Enjoy.

Jesus, pull my shirt tail when my self-righteousness heads in Martha's direction. You know the work to be done. Forgive me for acting as though I must do it all, especially when I am afraid it may be done without me. Thank you for my capacity for self-renewal, and bless my steps in that direction. Amen.

Intercedite pro Nobis

When the old customs and prayers "hit the spot"

Omnes sancti et sanctae Dei, intercedite pro nobis. All holy men and women, intercede for us.

Litany of the Saints

One day after a foreboding preliminary diagnosis and before the surgery which revealed that the condition was benign, I received a small Special Delivery package from my close friend, Su. An ordained Presbyterian minister, she was looking for a memento that would remind me of her prayers for me during this time of crisis. "Do you have anything for sick people?" she asked the proprietor of the local Catholic religious goods store. For an answer, he drew from behind the counter a chart that listed a comprehensive array of various ills and misfortunes, each with its own patron saint. "My stars!" she told me later. "With all those, I thought there might be one specifically for ovaries. Evidently there's just one saint who covers all cancers." Inside the box was a medal depicting Saint Peregrine. It required a concerted effort at the Duke Divinity School Library to discover that Peregrine was a thirteenth-century Servite priest who founded a monastery in Italy and whose grotesque foot cancer was cured by his trust in God's healing power.

It has been many, many years since I operated out of my early childhood belief that God was absolutely bound by the commonly held equations between prayer formulas and results. For example, as a child, I devoutly marked each November the Portiuncula indulgence, when, we believed, the recitation of fifteen Our Fathers, Hail Marys, and Glory Bes within the doors of a Catholic church would release one soul from purgatory. Catholic churches were filled with the faithful, who clustered just inside the doors so they could move in and out quickly, one soul each visit. Now, while my head suspects the skies were not filled with flocks of newly freed souls heaven-bound, that image stays with me as part of the way I think of death and the afterlife.

My head to the contrary, one of my favorite parts of Catholicism is its earthy simplicity, its literalism, its myths. For instance, how do I know that God is right in here with me when I am so overwhelmed by the day's confusion that I lose everything I touch? Well, because there's Saint Anthony. Again, my head says that seven Glory Bes said in petition followed quickly by seven in thanksgiving (so Saint Anthony will feel beholden if he doesn't find the lost article) do not weave a compelling web around God or my car keys.

No, but I do know something even more important than that. I know that nothing about my life is insignificant before God. And I know that God is with me even in the frazzled times; that another name for God's practical providential protection of me is Christopher; that God is with me as surely as with Peregrine in times of sickness; that God will help me to be steadfast and clearsighted in the midst of conflicting values as in the Saint Lucy legend, that God speaks to the church through strong women because the heroines of the Catherine, Teresa, and Hildegard stories spoke volumes; and that the bonds among the people of God unite both the living and the dead we prayed for during the Portiuncula indulgence period.

Dear God, while your presence sometimes seems impossibly nebulous, you've peopled the world of our faith with whole cities of saints whose stories capture who you are in the flesh. While I sometimes smile at old Catholic trivia, I thank you for the truth of these legends, and for your care for me that reaches into every corner of my life. Amen.

11

Worry About Clothing?

When your own worries seem trifling

And why do you worry about clothing? Consider the lilies of the field, how they grow; they neither toil nor spin,
yet I tell you, even Solomon in all his glory was not
clothed like one of these.   Matthew 6:28

This morning, I underwent a medical procedure which, in the
global scheme of things, was definitely relatively minor. But it
seemed big to me. And it was drawn out and painful, not to
mention isolating, in the white-and-stainless-steel radiology
room. Midway, when I thought my threshold of pain had
probably been violated quite enough, thank you, I thought of
praying. But I couldn't/didn't, thinking shamefacedly of the
women on the bone marrow transplant unit upstairs, or the
mother of the new cystic fibrosis patient, or the recurring melanoma patients I had just left. What right had I to think I had
any claim to pray to God for strength to get through my trifling pain, in the face of their far greater need!

Now, tonight, when the day is over and the responsibilities
that mercifully absorbed my attention after I left the clinic are
laid to rest, I remember my panic of this morning, and am
comforted by the sense of myself as one of the lilies of the
field. It is completely irrelevant that they "do not toil nor
spin," and I most certainly do. Tonight, I remembered that
God's care for all creation extends to me, toiling and spinning

away. And it encompasses me even when I don't or can't spin. Tonight, that Gospel vignette reminded me that I am never insignificant to God.

It strikes me that as caregivers, one of our occupational hazards is our concentrated exposure to life's most difficult and painful moments. We spend hours of our time moving close in to others' helplessness, pain, isolation, mortality, bitterness. For instance, the parish bulletin includes a wish list for some of the seemingly endless procession of desperately needy who spoke to our parish staff this week. The Eucharistic Minister who brought Communion to my home during my convalescence mused, "It's good to see someone who is going to get well." He was touched, I suspect, by the magnitude of some of the needs he witnesses each day as part of his ministry.

Sometimes that intensity comes as a blessing. This morning, I was ready to commit mayhem because I discovered a moldy sandwich in my son's underwear drawer *after* he cheerfully claimed to have cleaned his room. There's nothing like a busy day of visiting sick children and parents to put that incident in perspective.

The liability occurs when we develop our own brand of "survivor's guilt," feeling that our needs, problems, and fears are insignificant. In comparison with the immediacy and magnitude of the difficulties we see in the lives of those we serve, they may seem too small to pray about. In fact, viewed on the whole, one could gain the impression from the Gospels that in order to get God's attention, one must be either very sick or very bad. The chances are that, on a daily basis, we fit in neither category.

Still, we worry, hurt, regret, mourn, and storm against things in our own lives, not to mention the lives of our patients, parishioners, family members, and others we care for. And there it is, in Matthew. Even the birds of the air are fed by our heavenly Father; "Are you not of more value than they?" Jesus gently reminds his disciples (6:26). "But if God so clothes the grass of the field...will he not much more clothe you...? ...indeed your heavenly Father knows that you need all these things" (Matthew 6:30-32).

Dear Companion, it is good to know that you are there, even when my problems seem so small in comparison with others' needs that I am ashamed of my worry. Remind me, especially in those moments, that you will never abandon me. And then, open my eyes anew to the beauty of your world, which stands as a daily reminder of your abiding care. Amen.

12

Ten Made Clean

When your caregiving seems thankless

Then Jesus asked, "Were not ten made clean? But the other nine, where are they? Was none of them found to return and give praise to God except this foreigner?"
Luke 17:17

If anyone will not welcome you or listen to your words, shake off the dust from your feet as you leave that house or town.
Matthew 10:14

Several years ago, I was paged by two nurses who were at the bedside of an elderly comatose patient who was in the process of dying. They had cared for the gentleman for a long time—long enough to become attached, they said—and knew he had no one to be with him as he died. They had come to care about him, and wanted to be with him at this time. And they wanted a chaplain to be with the three of them. Together, we stood around his bed as his thin chest rose and fell in gradually lengthening intervals. The two nurses reminisced about their time with the patient, about his cheerfulness, quiet dignity, and gentleness. Finally, his breathing stopped. One of the nurses lifted her stethoscope to listen for a heartbeat, and the other went to call for a doctor to verify the death. When she returned, we had prayer, they each held one of his hands and tenderly kissed his forehead, then drew up the sheets preliminary to the morgue attendant's arrival.

Subsequently, the nurses thanked me for responding to their call. In truth, the experience was one that the three of us treasured, a duty we felt was supremely important. The task of providing companionship to this kind gentleman on his final journey was one we felt privileged in performing. But it did put me in mind later on of the other caretaking tasks I regularly perform without words of thanks that I can understand, and sometimes without any significant sense of meaning or accomplishment.

Now, as documentation, procedures, and statistical reports become more important in hospitals and other care-providing agencies as well, it occurs to me that we may find ourselves performing an increasing number of functions that seem thankless, irrelevant, time-consuming, and annoying. Before I succumb to cynicism, "shake off the dust," and move on, however, I find myself wondering if I am sensitive to the ways in which my ministry *is* effective, where seed does take root in fertile soil.

This is an opportunity to count the ways in which our service is received, in whatever vernacular. I think of the feisty elderly diabetic who seemed merely to tolerate my daily visits. Finally, at our last visit before he left the hospital, he voiced his struggle to find some Scripture that would justify his feeling helped by me, since his ecclesiology did not admit of women ministers. Rarely have I received a thank you that rasped on so many of my rough edges, but I was deeply touched as well.

The most difficult type of visit for me is the door-to-door introductory visit that so often involves what seems like no more than the exchange of pleasantries. Whereas I am energized by longer, more intense visits, these sap my energy. But when I am tempted to forego them, I remember my own experience as a patient, when the chaplain's brief introductory visit served as a reminder to me of the care of the people of God at a time when I was too anxious to talk.

A nurse commented to me recently about one of my student chaplains, "So often we are too busy to talk, but seeing Sue on the floor so often reminds us that she is available if we need her, and that she cares about us as well as the patients. That really helps." I suspect that Sue was unaware of the gratitude of the staff simply for her presence.

In reflecting on affirmation and thanks, I am reminded of how meaningful it has been to pass on positive feedback to others. The dietary staff was pleased when I shared my appreciation of their sensitivity about interrupting my visits with patients, for instance. It was an entirely new experience for the Housekeeping Department when several of us attended a departmental meeting to give our feedback on the impact of their cheerfulness and sensitivity to patients.

Dear Lord, my leader, I am sometimes more conscientious about following your call than sensitive to the rewards it offers. Open my heart to those simple, human ways in which my ministry is received and appreciated. Remind me to share my appreciation with others, as well. Amen.

13

Gathers Her Brood

When you are hurt by others' pain

Jerusalem, Jerusalem...how often have I desired to gather
your children together as a hen gathers her brood under
her wings....   Matthew 23:37

I used to be suspicious when patients attributed their feelings
to global issues—"The news is so depressing today," "Isn't it
awful about what happened...?" "How can there be such tragedy...?" Hearing that, I generally prepared myself to hone in
on or at least to be attentive to issues that struck closer to home
for them: personal loss, grief, pain of separation, new awareness of limitations, fragility, or mortality, for instance. After
all, it is often easier to deal with painful or difficult issues
"over there" than with those that touch us personally.

Lately, I've begun to rethink that. When a recent series of
events put me in touch more closely than usual with my own
mortality, I found myself tugged by something that felt larger
than my own condition. I remembered Gerard Manley
Hopkins's exquisite poem, "Spring and Fall," which describes
a young girl's melancholy as she watches golden leaves fall in
a favorite grove of trees. Hopkins attributes her sadness to the
finiteness and transitoriness of creation, as well as to her own
mortality as part of creation:

It is the blight man was born for,
It is Margaret you mourn for.*

One liability of our work, close as it is to illness, accident, tragedy and chaos, is that it may cause us to retreat inward, away from the harm we see so often. For instance, I spent one night helping two families deal with the deaths of their teen-aged son and daughter in an auto accident where speed and alcohol were involved. The next morning, I could hardly let my son leave for school; while I recognized the irrationality of my fears, it was hard to allow him out of my sight.

And yet, it seems important to maintain the wide view, to move out of our self-protectiveness, illusory as it is. I had to re-alize that I cannot protect my son forever, even from himself when he is irresponsible or immature. Further, I cannot protect myself from this kind of pain, if I seriously enter into the role of parent, minister, or other type of caregiver. Ultimately, my exposure to that pain as I empathize with those I serve sen-sitizes me to its inevitability and universality. "It is the blight...."

Perhaps that is the message of the second Beatitude: "Blessed are those who mourn, for they will be comforted" (Matthew 5:4). Commentaries apply that blessing both to those who had no worldly comfort and to those who mourned the status of the nation of Israel. In our ministry, we witness the individual tragedies in the lives of those who cannot easily be comforted. That calls us to an awareness of the suffering of the world, as people everywhere struggle with the wars, natural disasters, and painful limitations that are an inescapable part of being human. Sensitized to their individual griefs, our role

---

*W.H. Gardner and N.H. MacKenzie, eds. *The Poems of Gerard Manley Hopkins*. 4th ed. (New York: Oxford University Press, 1967), n. 55.

as ministers to the people of God draws us beyond those moments to concern and prayer for all creation.

Dear Lord, sometimes my work leaves me sad and heartsick almost beyond comfort. I know I've opened myself to that in accepting your call to this role. Nevertheless, it is often painful and frightening. Help me not to flee into whatever false security I can find, and draw me close beneath your comforting wings. Amen.

14

At Your House

When you perform sacramental ministry

When Jesus came to the place [where Zacchaeus had climbed in order to see him], he looked up and said to him, "Zacchaeus, hurry up and come down; for I must stay at your house today."   Luke 19:5

I think sometimes the beauty or perhaps simply the old familiarity of rituals helps us to be faithful even at those times when God seems capricious or malevolent or absent. I remember the times of my own tears of loneliness, fear, weariness, or futility. Add to that the questions raised by patients and families when their burdens and tragedies seem beyond bearing. I sometimes wonder where—and even if—God is.

And yet, I don't question the meaning of many of the old rituals I grew up with in the church. For example, the way that Communion was brought to the sick in Catholic hospitals. As a nurse's aide during my high school years, I remember kneeling in the hall or standing silently in the shadow of a doorway at the sound of the elevator door opening and the small bell ringing, often before dawn. First would come one of the Sisters with a candle and the bell. The priest would follow her, sweeping quickly through each room where the call light indicated the patient would like to receive Communion. All of us would wait in respectful silence until his pilgrimage through the unit was complete and the elevator door closed behind him.

Sometimes that ritual helps me to connect with my faith when reflection alone doesn't help. This is particularly true on those days when I spend a lot of my time away from patients or students, finishing paperwork or attending meetings that seem removed from "frontline ministry." It's a task I treasure, bringing Communion to some of the Catholic patients. I find myself quieting as I move to the hospital chapel to get a pyx, and then walk through the complex to the patient areas.

At those times, God's presence seems so tangible that I am startled when friends greet me as usual; it must be obvious to all, I think, that I have Someone with me. "Make ready the way of the Lord," I shout inside. I expect that "even the stones will cry out" in reply. I fantasize about interrupting those who run through the halls, bent over with hurried intensity. "Wait a moment," I cry. "The Lord is here, in our hospital. Come down, medical center Zacchaeuses! Let's celebrate, or rest a moment with him, or say directly whatever is on our minds. We can speak up; he has come to spend some time with us." My imagination runs ahead of me when I board the patient elevator, crowded with gurneys. "Just a second," I think I say. "I have Someone with me who can grant you anything you wish; what'll it be? Successful surgery? Complete remission? A cure? You've got it!"

I'm probably a good bit safer in patient rooms, but even there, my exuberance abounds. My greeting, "I've brought you Communion, if you would like to receive today," is met promptly as patients and visitors close magazines, interrupt conversations, and cross themselves. Together we chorus through the ritual of Communion of the Sick, I distribute the hosts, and leave. I wonder if their sense of being visited is as tangible as it seems to me.

When my circuit is complete, my part of the Catholic patient list visited, I return to the chapel. I am reluctant, and have new sensitivity to Peter's impulsive gesture at the Transfiguration: "Master, it is good for us to be here; let us make three dwellings..." (Luke 9:33). It *is* hard to leave the mountain.

Dearest Lord, don't be such a stranger! Thank you so much for those moments when your presence seems tangible, when believing is joyful and freeing, and when our ministry is clearly and sensibly a blessed privilege. Amen.

15

Remove This Cup

When you are faced with difficult decisions

And going a little farther, he threw himself on the ground
and prayed that, if it were possible, the hour might pass
from him. He said, "Abba, Father, for you all things are
possible; remove this cup from me; yet, not what I want,
but what you want."   Mark 14:35-36

"Unfortunately, it's a trade off," mused the medical team die-
titian in a discussion of a rare children's digestive disorder.
"The kids who do the best physically have controlling mothers
who watch every bite they eat. But they're the kids who then
can't grow into normal adolescent independence. Conversely,
the ones who develop best emotionally do the worst physically
because they make their own decisions—and they often don't
observe their dietary restrictions."

How seldom medical decisions are clearcut these days.
Antibiotics may cure a minor sore throat now, but with con-
tinued use, the body may develop an immunity rendering
them useless against more serious infections later. "Miracle
drugs" may have side effects that are more disabling than the
original problem they were invented to treat. More and more
frequently, physicians present patients and families with a
menu of possible treatments and outcomes from which they
must choose. How painful are these dilemmas! And the decision process itself: While patients and family members long

for control, there are times when it might seem easier if someone else made those decisions for them. "Doctor, what do *you* think we should do?" they plead. "Please tell us!"

As care providers, however, we notice and probably applaud the trend toward choices and patients' rights to decide. Still, I recently heard one physician declare that there are many situations where he does not present alternatives to his patients. When he doubts their ability to make "correct" choices, he makes the decisions himself. While many of us took issue with what sounded dangerously like paternalism, we could all remember cases where it might have been much easier on all involved to forego discussion.

As caregivers, we witness countless situations like these. I suspect that it is easier to sense God's presence when outcomes are either inevitable or totally unpredictable. For example, cancer patients and their families frequently come to a place where they acknowledge that it is time for death, and that dying would be a blessing. Or with heart surgery that could as easily result in restoration of health as in death, there is usually no question about which way to pray.

But it is most difficult to sense God's care when there are decisions to be made. Scripture attests to the pain of those moments. For instance, Jesus is very clear to the Rich Young Man about his choices: "If you wish to be perfect, go, sell your possessions, and give the money to the poor, and you will have treasure in heaven; then come, follow me" (Matthew 19:21). Although the fellow has already directed his life toward good ("Teacher, I have kept all these [commandments] since my youth," Mark 10:20), this further step is too difficult. Nevertheless, his decision is not an easy one: "When the young man heard this word, he went away grieving, for he had many possessions" (Matthew 19:22). Or the calling of the disciples: While the invitations and acceptances appear to have been fairly straightforward and uncomplicated, it is Peter who reminds Jesus that those decisions may not have been so easily made. "Then Peter said in reply, 'Look, we have left everything and followed you. What then will we have?'" (Matthew 19:27). Or Jesus' own choices in the desert: Jesus seems to have no hesitation in rejecting each of the devil's proposals. The fact that "The devil left him, and suddenly angels came and waited on him," would seem to indicate that the confrontation required energy.

As much as we wish for control, then, decision making is a two-edged sword. Those moments place us in the driver's seat, at least for some of the journey. But they also confront us with the consequences of our choices. And sometimes, the best decision in the world cannot bring about a happy ending.

Dearest Lord, it is sometimes so easy to feel your presence. At times, the sense of being held and supported by you is almost tangible. We thank you for the times when things are going well. But even more today, we ask for your peace during this time of decision. Help us to make careful, wise choices, or to minister to those in our care who must make difficult decisions today. But most of all, help us to remember that you are always with us, even when the answers and the courses of action seem unclear to us. Amen.

16

What Do You Say?

When you are tempted to judge

The scribes and the Pharisees brought a woman who had
been caught in adultery; and making her stand before all
of them, they said to him, "Teacher, this woman was
caught in the very act of committing adultery. In the law
Moses commanded us to stone such women. Now what
do you say?"   John 8:4,5

At first glance, it was easy to take sides. Six-year-old Josh had
been hospitalized most of a year with a brain tumor. Karen, his
mother, moved into his hospital room to care for him, while
Bob, his father, immersed himself in his work. As Josh's condition worsened, Bob's visits became less frequent, and Karen's
anger increased. In Bob's absence, the staff sided with Karen.
In my pastoral visits, she focused on her apprehension about
her future without Josh, and her anger with her husband. My
attempts to meet with him were fruitless. When Josh died, it
was Karen who told me what she wished for his funeral, and it
was she who met me before the service to reminisce and pray
together at his bier.

So it caught me by surprise, when, as the mourners left the
service to go to the cemetery, Bob asked me to remain behind
with him for a moment. I followed him silently, as he ap-
proached the coffin with a paper sack and drew out a thread-
bare blanket and teddy bear. Then, tearfully and with

incredible tenderness, he tucked his son in for the last time, kissed his forehead, and closed the casket. There were no words to be said. And for the first time, I understood with my heart the reason for his absence during those months.

Later, I reflected on how common it is for families in times of stress to fragment, for members to withdraw when the pain at their center seems too great to bear together. Even more, how easy it is to take sides, to assign blame. As caregivers, it is inevitable that we hear those "sides." "My sisters haven't done anything to help Mom; the load is all on me." "I don't think that nurse likes me; she won't answer my light." "That patient's family is not supportive; they rarely visit him." "Mom, make Jimmy stop hitting me!" And often (unless Jimmy is close behind) we hear only one side. It's so easy to move from empathy to commiserating with the person in front of us at the moment.

Yet, as I continue to learn, there are two sides to every issue. When I forget that, I find that my very wish to help sometimes gets me in trouble. When I move past empathy, I run the risk of leaving myself open to being manipulated ("Jimmy, leave your sister alone and go to your room!") as soon as I take sides. Or my judgment can easily be skewed, limited to the view of the person who has my ear. Most important, it seems to me, is that both sides generally need care. Given the logistics of health care facilities, we may not ever meet the "other side." But when we do, reaching out to them is easier if we haven't already judged them. For instance, would our efforts to involve Bob have been more effective if we had reached to his grief rather than blamed his absence?

Our pastoral and/or caregiving role affords us the luxury of not having to make judgments. In fact, our most valuable contribution may be our ability to look for and to minister to all sides.

Jesus, you have placed me at many temple squares, where I hear countless stories about broken relationships, hurt feelings, unmet obligations. Make me sensitive to the pain that flows through all the fragments. May I be a channel of your tenderness and understanding to all. Give me your strength and patience when I reach my own limits. Amen.

17

All Who Are Weary

When you need a good friend

Come to me, all you that are weary and are carrying
heavy burdens, and I will give you rest.   Matthew 11:28

It happened again, leaving me feeling irritated and used. An
acquaintance I hadn't heard from in months called late at
night, waking me from a sound sleep. Remembering our close-
ness in the past, I listened as she brought me up to date on her
recent difficulties and setbacks. I empathized with her frustration in single parenting her teenaged son and her depression at
facing an empty nest before too much longer. At length, she
reached a stopping point, paused, and asked about me. I began
to tell her about a decision I had recently made. "Why on earth
would you ever do that?" she interrupted. "Well, hon, I've got
to run." With that, she hung up, leaving me wide awake and
feeling out of joint.

Lately, I've been reflecting on the occupational hazards of
caregiving. I've begun to wonder if we're not better at taking
care of others than in connecting with friends who can care for
us in more balanced relationships of mutual giving and receiving. Of course, I'm not speaking of the kind of selflessness

that undergirds the ministry of caregiving in any arena. Rather, I'm thinking of habitual self-abnegation, where one gives to others either because one feels unworthy to receive or because one hopes eventually to earn care in return.

My sense is that caregivers' skills often flow out of their own painful history. For instance, my daughter's keen intuition about others' hurt has been shaped by her own past as a refugee and war survivor. How many nurses, social workers, and chaplains come from dysfunctional backgrounds such as alcoholic families? My faith leads me to believe that God redeems that pain by calling us to minister to others, sensitized to their need by our awareness of our own needs and pain. The problem is that we may never get around to our own needs in a straightforward way that renews us and replenishes our resources. Or our past may have led us to feel unworthy of being cared for, listened to, treated with warmth and regard.

I've learned to be suspicious of those caregivers who seem without needs or limits, without boundaries around their private time and lives, and without healthy friends who can give nurture, empathy, and an occasional reality check. We can take vicarious delight in Jesus' reassurance to Peter, "Come on, you *can* walk on water," and in Peter's acceptance and trust of his friend's affirmation. When we're tired, we can remember Jesus' taking time away from the crowds for rest and prayer (Matthew 14:23), or for a post-resurrection beach fish fry (John 21:4-14). Jesus did not think it a waste of time, attention, or money to allow his head to be anointed with costly lotion by the woman at the feast at the house of Simon (Matthew 26:10-13). Remembering those moments helps us to take time for ourselves, and to draw closer to those friends in our lives who are willing and able to nurture us when we need care.

Jesus, you know how much I love to help people. I take satisfaction in speaking your healing word of comfort and consolation to those in pain or need. Make me as sensitive to my own needs as I am to the needs of others. Help me to be honest in taking good care of myself. Surround me with good friends, and teach me to accept their love and care graciously and with enjoyment. Amen.

18

He Went Away

When you wish you could control others

Jesus said to him, "If you wish to be perfect, go, sell your possessions...then come, follow me." When the young man heard this word, he went away grieving, for he had many possessions. Matthew 19:21,22

On a recent blazing hot summer day, my son and I walked to a nearby shopping center. As we neared our destination, we found ourselves being "buzzed" by two landlocked sandpipers. At the shore, their staccato march back and forth in the surf is entertaining. But here, they shrieked frantically as they alternately dived at our heads and flopped awkwardly on the hot pavement. Gradually we noticed the reason for their worry. Three stairstep fledglings, ranging from tiny ball of fluff to half grown, had scattered in all directions, and were determinedly foiling their parents' best and loudest efforts to corral them. My son and I joined the roundup. For a time, that only excited the little ones and confused the parents. Finally we managed to capture the offspring and move them to a shaded strip of grass and bushes. After all that work, I half expected some sign of relief or rest from the adult sandpipers. Not so. They flew off to continue their squawking and pacing on another corner of the parking lot. And on our return, the fledglings were gone without a trace.

None of my reflections on the incident had to do with the worry- and toil-free life of birds, who, as Jesus tells the story, "neither sow nor reap." In fact, I had a good bit more empathy for them than envy, as I turned to see my own offspring vanish into traffic. What did occur to me was how difficult and complicated caregiving can be. What does it mean to be responsible for a child or aging parent who is, in my mother's vernacular, "independent as a hog on ice"? In health care, patient autonomy is an increasingly important value, as we struggle to do well by patients even when that involves educating and empowering them to the point where they may sometimes discard our advice. As a shepherd, when do I follow my lambs through the stormy dark far pasture to bear them back from danger, and when do I "simply" issue warnings about the dangers as I see them?

The path to an answer—if there is one—is further complicated by the paradox that those we care for often intuitively know what kind of care they need. At the least, they know what kind of care they will accept. *Our* very best informed and most caring interventions are sometimes erroneous or inadequate...or ignored. So while we scurry frantically around and through our children's, parents', and patients' needs, they may fend us off and then fly off gracefully on their own.

We generally think of the Ministry of Presence as focusing on empathy, on reaching out to those we serve in the midst of their struggles and conflicts without distracting ourselves about finding the right words or saying the right things. My musings on the sandpipers have led me to suspect that an equally difficult aspect of the Ministry of Presence is listening intently to others' thoughts and plans without becoming distracted and carried away by my wishes and plans for them, without giving my advice and sharing my experience prematurely. Somehow, that sounds easy. In practice? Well, I really wanted to tell those sandpipers that if they had built their nest in a sensible place....

Dearest Lord, perhaps it is because there are so few absolute answers and guarantees in the work of caregiving that I embrace with enthusiasm those times when I am sure my answer is right or that my advice will make a difference to those I love and care for. Give me the prudence to know when my advice is appropriate, and the wisdom to know how to blend support and silence. Amen.

19

Walking on the Water

When you encounter risks

Peter answered him, "Lord, if it is you, command me to come to you on the water." He said, "Come." So Peter got out of the boat, started walking on the water, and came toward Jesus.   Matthew 14:28,29

A number of years ago, I traveled through Reno with a friend on our way to summer school. We had agreed beforehand to limit our gambling to four dollars each. She won a small fortune in quarters. I, unwilling to risk even four dollars, bought myself some orange juice—the only sure bet in the city.

So I feel a bit bad each new semester when I talk to new chaplain students about our kind of caregiving. When you get right down to it, each discipline in a health care facility has its tools of the trade. Respiratory therapists have airways and oxygen tanks. Surgeons have scalpels and sutures. Nurses have stethoscopes and charts, and lab technicians have their collections of tubes and needles.

And what do we have? Our faith, and our sensitivity to our own and others' feelings and spiritual values. That's it. That's ^ *risk!*

And, while risk is sometimes thrilling and exhilarating, it isn't always all it's cracked up to be. That's why I find a sort of vicarious excitement in following Peter's odyssey through the

Gospels. Peter—the recipient of some of Jesus' hardest words. Peter—sometimes flippant, often slow to learn, invariably speaking the lines we would say—if we had the nerve...if we could risk.

"You are the salt of the earth...you are the light of the world" (Matthew 5:13,14), Peter and the other apostles are told, and we can feel sometimes the weariness that goes with the responsibilities of faithfulness, of shepherding and supporting those who look to us for witness. Peter is the challenger, the asker of questions. "Look, we have left everything and followed you. What then will we have?" (Matthew 19:28) he confronts Jesus. Or, "My God! How many times am I supposed to forgive this brother of mine?" (Matthew 18:21) "Look, Lord, this 'blind leading the blind' parable—it doesn't make good sense. Explain it to us" (Matthew 15:15). Finally, Jesus knows who among the group he can count on for the perfect opening; he knows that Peter can risk being his "straight man." And so while it is to all of the apostles that he addresses his question, "Who do *you* say I am?" it is Peter who risks the perfect answer, "You are the Messiah, the Son of the living God" (Matthew 16:16).

I admit that I might have had a second thought before answering so quickly, if I had been there. It's hard to risk. It's hard to be told that one's pastoral role will sometimes entail being sent forth like sheep among wolves (Matthew 10:16), like healthy caregivers among the sick. It's hard to feel cold water lapping at your toes—and then your knees. I fantasize sometimes that Peter returns to the place of his walk on the water to try it again. It is surely a fitting reward for such a risk to find that one can stay afloat, exhilarated by the wind and waves, successfully buoyed by faith.

Dear Jesus, our leader and model for ministry, you call us to many difficult and frightening tasks. So much of the time, we enjoy the service we are able to give. Give us strength in those times when the risk of service to others and of looking into ourselves in order to know how to reach others seems costly and painful. Remind us of the strength we can find in you and in the community of faith. Amen.

20

The Valley of the Weeper

When you can care for yourself

Happy those whose strength is in you; they have courage
to make the pilgrimage! As they go through the Valley of
the Weeper, they make it a place of springs, clothed in
generous growth by early rains.   Psalm 84:5-6*

Dr. Oliver Sacks, the neurologist-model for the movie
Awakenings, once described his own experience as a patient in
a convalescent home. There, he noticed an unexpected lightness among the patients despite their pain. "An outsider
would have thought us a frivolous lot," he wrote. "...If we
were frivolous, it was the high spirits of the newborn—and
equally of those who have known the deepest darkness." Our
contribution to those in our care is our willingness to empathize with their pain. But this also poses a hazard to our
own health and balance, when we are unable to find hope or
meaning in their lives or in ours either. In his analysis of the
poetry of Gerard Manley Hopkins, Donald Walhout** describes the cycles of spiritual desolation Hopkins experienced
during much of his adult life, as well as the phases through
which he moved out of them. It occurred to me that his resources for recovery were as common and accessible as the
Psalmist's "early rains." Nevertheless, they bear mentioning,

---

*Nancy Schreck, OSF and Maureen Leach, OSF, *Psalms Anew* (Winona, Minn.:
Saint Mary's Press, 1986).
**Send My Roots Rain* (Athens, Ohio: Ohio University Press, 1981).

especially for those of us who sometimes lose ourselves in what Sacks called "deepest darkness."

For Hopkins, the list of natural wellsprings of spiritual healing and rebirth includes these: nature, beauty, creative activity, moral resolve, ability to do daily work, human association, spiritual discipline, and humor. When we are sad or discouraged or demoralized, it is difficult to imagine that those feelings could be dissipated easily. Nevertheless, all of us have experienced being startled out of a painful mood by an unexpected view of the sunset, or a call from a friend, the satisfaction of completing a task, the getting back into a familiar routine after a time of disruption, or a really good laugh. We remember the satisfaction we derive from investing ourselves in causes we believe in, and in seeing the good we can accomplish. Or hobbies, where we can forget our mood in the delight of watching a needlepoint pattern emerge or a garden take shape and produce food and flowers we enjoy.

In the end, renewal through these natural means is one stage in our process of becoming increasingly aware of God's faithful presence in creation, in our lives, despite our discouragement or fatigue, and in the lives of those we serve, despite the trials with which they struggle.

Lord, sometimes it feels disloyal or frivolous to be joyful and happy in the face of the pain, sorrow, and limitations in the lives of those we minister to. I am grateful for the ways in which your creation leads me to you, and for the joy that draws me closer to your goodness. Thank you for refreshment that comes to me through the beauty of the earth and the activities I enjoy. Help me to see them as evidence of your presence and love for me. Amen.

21

God's Seal

When you are ordained by those you serve

It is God who establishes us with you in Christ and has
anointed us, by putting his seal on us and giving us his
Spirit in our hearts as a first installment....you are a letter
of Christ...written not with ink but with the Spirit of the
living God, not on tablets of stone but on tablets of human hearts.   2 Corinthians 1:21-2:2,3

In the ecclesiastical kingdom of my childhood, the parish pastor was regent. The stairway to the throne was shrouded in
mystery, and celebrated in rituals which we revered but were
not a part of. What a contrast with the contemporary Rite of
Christian Initiation, where new members are prepared for
their role as priestly people. In countless parishes, this theme
threads through all the sacramental preparation programs, as
candidates focus on both doctrinal formation and service as
components of their membership. For their part, congregation
members participate in the rituals by promising their prayers
and concrete support of the candidates.

The importance of that theme as it operates for caregivers is
sometimes overlooked, given the church's dearth of significant
rituals marking the ministry of lay chaplains, religious ed-

ucators, and other relatively new ministerial roles. However, that lack behooves us to pay greater attention to the less "official" but no less important rituals marking our ministry.

Ritual is a language of familiar word and gesture that communicates important meanings within a community. I've thought of my own ordination as occurring nearly ten years ago, when the son of a comatose patient whom I had visited for weeks noticed the damage hospital soap had done to my hands, and anointed them with Dermassage from his mother's bedside stand before we prayed together. I've treasured that moment. His gesture empowered my ministry far beyond the reach of secular job descriptions and contracts.

I suspect that comparable ordination rituals occur many times each day, if we are attuned to the language. Given his choice of evening prayers, my son invariably asks for a "Mother's Blessing," thus ordaining me to bring closure to one day and hope for the next. Similar commissionings occur in the simplest gestures—a patient's making room for me to sit down in her room, conveying her wish that I would spend some time pastoring her, for instance. A nurse's apology, "I'm sorry for interrupting your conversation; I'll come back," is an acknowledgment of my ministry. Chaplains' inclusion on every Code team is recognition of our service to patients, family, and staff in critical situations. In teaching institutions, the length of one's uniform coat is a status symbol. In our discipline, this is a badge of our service, comparable to the priest's stole. My handwashing before entering a patient's room and the priest's handwashing at Mass strike me as similar preparations for Jesus' presence in special ways "where two or more are gathered" in his name. These are the "words" of our ordination, for those who can hear.

Dear Lord, amid the fireworks of your more spectacular miracles and wonders is your reliance on the common stuff of daily routine—water, wine, bread, washing, reaching out a hand, feeding....Draw my attention to the significance of the simple pieces of my work and their meaning in my ministry to your people. Amen.

22

Come Out

When those we serve call us forth

Jesus cried out with a loud voice, "Lazarus, come out!"
The dead man came out, his hands and feet bound with
strips of cloth, and his face wrapped in a cloth. Jesus said
to them, "Unbind him, and let him go."   John 11:44

One assumption undergirding much of the practice of pastoral
care is that it is helpful for people in stress or need to talk
about their feelings, and that doing this in a religious context
helps the recipients to bring their own spiritual resources to
bear on their situation. My own second assumption is that as
the "caregiver," I am also the recipient of the wisdom they've
won as they thread their way through universal human experiences that I haven't had yet. I minister by listening to their
stories unfold and by receiving their witness. They minister to
me by helping me to prepare for my own encounters with unexpected, out of control, painful, even mystical eventualities.

From that stance, I've wondered what Lazarus must have
told his sisters about his experience of dying and coming back.
I have some hunches, having listened to others at crossroads
between life and death or between life-as-usual and some in-
tervening circumstance. For instance, I wonder how his experience affected his sense of proportion. We have some
evidence that Mary, Martha, and Lazarus had their stormy moments; what did they consider worth quarreling about after his

return to life? What kinds of things upset him? What did he lose sleep over, after his resurrection?

How did his experience affect relationships? What do our patients tell us about relationships? "My brothers and sisters were never close," said one patient to me yesterday. "I'm not sure if they'd come to be with me now, but I'm going to ask." Another patient and Family Hero reflected on her role and the anger she drew from it, and began to ask other family members to assume more responsibility for tasks she could no longer perform. Listening to her, I looked at my propensity for self-righteous busyness.

Use of time? We've all heard reflections like, "I would (will) take more time for little things." I used to take pride in how fast I could sprint from one meeting to another throughout the hospital where I minister. When I returned to work after a recent illness, I first realized that for a while, at least, I could not sprint. I also realized that I no longer wanted to, that I lose the centeredness that undergirds my joy as well as my effectiveness when I rush from one activity to another that way. One grace-ful result of my own "Lazarus" experience was that I plan ten minutes for "travel time" between meetings now.

What did Lazarus learn about spiritual struggles and their resolution? In retrospect, one of the things that surprises me about the deaths I've witnessed is that there has almost always been some sense of acceptance amid whatever anger, denial, grief, and pain may also be there. When I'm discouraged or sad, it is difficult to imagine that I may feel differently in the morning, next week, at the end of the semester. At other times, I get impatient over my own slowness in finding meaning or effecting change in my world. My patients have taught me much about the natural rhythm of the human body and spirit that finds wholeness and peace in its own best time.

What other messages would Lazarus have shared? What do those we care for tell us from their experience?

Dear Lord, you called forth Lazarus from the darkness of physical death and the tomb. With the voice of those I serve, you call me from the darkness of my own limited perspective. I thank you for the wisdom they share with me, and I ask for your strength as I strive to listen well and fearlessly to the lessons they teach me. Amen.

23

My Enemies

When your enemies are within

Be gracious to me, O God, for the enemy persecutes me; my adversaries harass me all day long...for you have rescued me from death—to walk in your presence, in the light of life.   Psalm 56:1,13

I've always been rather skeptical of the "drop the needle" approach to finding God's current directions for me in Scripture. So I had some theological adjustments to make when, after a particularly harrowing encounter with my mortality, I opened my Bible to Psalm 56.

It has also seemed a bit risky to label my enemies quite so blithely as the Psalmist seems to do, partly lest they similarly label me. But in order to accept the promise of new life in the second half of the Psalm, I had to take seriously the first half, the part that speaks about enemies. What struck me was that the enemies that militate most strongly against my entering into "new life" fully each day are those within me.

So with the Psalmist looking over my shoulder, I take inventory. There's one enemy I know well, the one that leads me to assume that my opinion is the best one, perhaps the only one. When the others in my life slow me down enough to hear theirs, I am often surprised at the differences in viewpoint. When no one slows me down....

My second enemy whispers the AA prayer about "changing

the things I can change, accepting the things I can't change, and having the wisdom to know the difference." I generally err in the direction of acceptance, neglecting to change the things I can and should change. I rush too much, pleading family demands. I use the same excuse for not taking time for myself, a step that carries considerably more risk than filling my life completely with the care of others.

Let's see. My third enemy provides me with lots of storage room for the bits and pieces of anger I've kept through the years. My enemies "out there" are not nearly so faithful as I in keeping them around. There was the time when she said...and he forgot...and we always...but they didn't....

How petty some of those enemies seem. And yet, how difficult it is to exorcize those demons, to clean out that attic of the accumulated junk. I am skeptical, even irritated, at the ease with which the Psalmist disposes of enemies described as so formidable (Psalm 56:6):

All day long they plot to harm me:
all their thoughts are hostile.
They are on the lookout:
they conspire and spy on my footsteps.

In a mere thirteen verses, such an enemy is "turned back," dispatched simply because the Psalmist calls on God (Psalm 56:10,11):

For this I know—that God is with me.
In God I trust and shall not be afraid.

Perhaps there is a lesson for us here. It is surprisingly easy for us to name the enemies that clutter our own souls, discouragingly difficult to clear them out. So don't worry about it! In my struggle to vanquish those enemies, I forget that it is God who does that. My role, according to the Psalmist, is to trust and not be afraid. Then, God brings ruin to them and new life to me.

Lord, sometimes we make things so complicated and difficult. Help us to trust that you know all about our enemies and battles, and that you will do your part in standing with us. And then help us to enjoy and to rest in your presence, in the light of life.

24

The Lord Called

When you can't sleep

Samuel was lying down in the temple of the Lord, where the ark of God was. Then the Lord called, "Samuel! Samuel!" and he said, "Here I am!"   1 Samuel 4:3,4

Several years ago, I volunteered as a test subject for a study on pain management. One of the techniques being tested was reframing. Instead of thinking, "How awful, my head aches," we were instructed to send ourselves positive messages like, "My head is taking care of me by telling me that I am tense, or need to change my position," etc.

Actually, headaches never got me down. But sleepless nights? That's another thing. In fact, I've wondered sometimes if sleeplessness might not be the occupational hazard of caregivers. Nothing disturbs a parent's sleep patterns on weekend nights as surely as having a teenager old enough to drive. Yesterday, a neighbor was telling me about the toll on her two aunts, as they take turns getting up at night to turn their bedridden mother. A co-worker describes her wakefulness with worry about her limit-testing son. Last night, I found myself jolted awake by the sudden remembering of a patient I promised to visit.

I used to be—and sometimes still am—resentful about those wakeful hours when I found it difficult to go to sleep, knowing how tired I would be in the morning. Frustrated and having nothing to lose by trying a new approach, I began to look at those minutes and hours as "found time," almost like an unexpected windfall of money that one gets to spend on something extra or frivolous for oneself.

Instead of tossing and turning or fretting away those hours, then, I began to use them for things I love to do but generally don't have time for. I rejected journaling during that time, because writing about my wakefulness kept me focused on my frustration. The same with writing letters to friends, unless I could get past, "Dear Liz, I couldn't sleep, so...."

No, my list of late night special activities tended toward items like these: 1) My supermarket magazine collection, issues I bought as an occasional splurge but never had time to read: I read any article that sounds interesting, including the makeover tips and miracle diet and exercise programs. 2) Hobby needlework, like the embroidery projects I find enjoyable and relaxing. Only recreational sewing; my personal "house rule" allows no mending after 9:00 at night. 3) Recreational reading, anything from "bodice-rippers" to mysteries. I've been working my way through the library's list of mysteries featuring women sleuths, for instance. 4) During my "found time," I slather on some "Passion" lotion, a special gift from a friend. If I'm still not sleepy, I give myself a manicure. 5) I rarely do "recreational cooking" any more, but I enjoy looking through my recipes and cookbooks. This is a good time for recalling occasions when I've made my favorites and for resolving to make them again. 6) I'm a flower pot gardener, but not even very dedicated to that. Nights are a quiet time to prune, re-pot, water, and rearrange my plants.

Paradoxically, giving myself the freedom to enjoy my wakefulness often helps me to drift off quickly, instead of fretting until I *am* wide awake.

Lord, you've startled your people with strange messages at strange times. Open my tired ears to your words to me when they come as I try to sleep. When I am anxious about gathering my energy for the work of tomorrow, awaken me to the simple pleasures I sometimes neglect in the frenzy of the day. And finally, bring me the gift of sleep. Amen.

25

One of the Least

When you are "one of the least"

And the king will answer them, "Truly I tell you, just as you did it to one of the least of these who are members of my family, you did it to me."   Matthew 25:40

As much as I've assumed the notion of God as transcendent, recently I've been most aware that God is revealed to me through other people. Further, it has struck me anew that God cares for me in the presence and gestures of other people. This is such an old familiar truth that it seems silly to speak of it as though it were a new discovery. But there are those times when God's transcendence seems like absence, at least from any concerns of ours. And it is especially at those moments that the kindness of others breaks in on our painful isolation in ways that seem nothing short of miraculous.

I was mulling this over with a friend the other day, after a period when I had felt frightened and alone. I had been startled when, in the midst of that physical and spiritual tangle, help both from friends and from people I hardly knew appeared nearly before I could ask. God's presence grew tangible in others' active concern. But then, that itself seemed like fragile comfort to me, that God's presence in an important way depends on our presence to one another. After all, what about the times that others don't come forth when I am in need, and when I am insensitive or unwilling to reach out to others?

"All the more reason to marvel," said my friend, "at the heroism of folks who each day, consciously or not, undertake the work of being God to those around them." That term, "heroism," caught my attention; I've been thinking about the quiet heros in my life ever since.

One of my heros ministered to me by worrying. It's rare, I suspect, that caregivers get worried about. They generally exude strength and competence, and during times of confusion or danger, *they* do the worrying. Parents try not to unload their worries on their children, for instance, and they definitely don't want their children worrying about them. I was touched, then, when an old friend said, "I was worried about you." Actually, I was worried, too, and it was affirming to have company. Then, even though I wasn't sure where God was at that time, I knew I wasn't alone.

Another of my heros is a shy CPE student. Few knew how much energy it cost him to knock on hospital door after door, taking the initiative to greet strangers. When we did notice his custom of addressing everyone he met by name, he revealed his technique for memorizing names. He felt this was an important part of his ministry. As much as my heart warms to my children's name for my role as Mama for them, others' calling me by the name of my person feels affirming to me. I think the importance of God's calling me by name wouldn't make much sense unless I had some experience of being similarly remembered and affirmed by other people.

When I was recently housebound for several Sundays, a parish Eucharistic Minister brought me Communion. I was determined not to let one ounce of my illness experience go unexplored for what God might be saying to me, and I probably sounded fairly desperate about my Search for Meaning at that point. Each week, Mary Ann brought Communion...and the

New York Times. She truly helped me to see that God could as easily speak to me if I enjoyed my recuperation. What a graceful hero she was for me.

Who are the people who embody God for you, who tell you in contemporary terms who God is?

Thank you, dear God, for your presence in burning bushes, in pillars of fire, in the rainbow, and most of all, in Jesus. I thank you especially for your presence here and now in those who reach out to me, who remind me by their honesty, kindness, practicality, and faithfulness of who you are in my life. Amen.

Of Related Interest...

Body, Mind & Spirit
To Harmony through Meditation
Louis Hughes

Simple exercises conducive to prayer that relax the body and mind while freeing the spirit. Practical examples show how meditation can free energy spent on nervousness and tension for more positive activities.
128 pp, $7.95

At Ease with Stress
Wanda Nash

Shows readers how to make stress work in their favor. Includes creative solutions to overcome stesss, including meditations and reflections.
224 pp, $9.95

From Worry to Wellness
21 People Who Changed Their Lives
Ruth Morrison and Dawn Radtke

Offers positive, practical ways to change for the better, based on real-life examples.
192 pp, $7.95

Seek Treasures in Small Fields
Everyday Holiness
Joan Puls

Encourages readers to tap into the "treasures" that lie beneath the "small fields" of everyday life experiences. Shows how to find the hidden significance in daily life.
160 pp, $7.95

Available at religious bookstores or from
TWENTY-THIRD PUBLICATIONS
P.O. Box 180 • Mystic, CT 06355 • 1-800-321-0411